D1824726

something beginning with me... at 21

First published in Great Britain in 2012 by
Something beginning with me - April 2012
ISBN - 978-0-9567112-5-0

Dedicated to Tom Hurley, Rae George & Liam Jones

Publisher: Something beginning with me Ltd
Web address: www.sbwm.co
e-mail: erica@sbwm.co

Cover design: So design consultants Ltd.
www.so-design.co.uk

Models in cover design: Tom Astley
www.tomastley.com

Something beginning with me...

How to use this book:

This book is for you to use like a diary, it will help you to record where you are as come of age. Looking at where you are starting and how you would like things to be, it is a place for you to write down your dreams, goals and ideas for your future.

It'll help you understand more about what's important to you, the things that you enjoy and the things that annoy you, helping you to explore the things that you'd like to carry on doing and the things you'd like to stop doing, to help you to get what you want...

You may have used another SBWM book, if you did, then you might want to look to see how you've changed and realise how much you have already achieved...

We all have things about ourselves that we like and other things that we would change if we could. Some of these things we cannot change, but for those that we can, we may need a little help and support to make sure we can achieve them.

This book is set out in chapters to will help you to look at how you feel about yourself and others and to help you to set some goals around these as you start your first real job. Most importantly there is plenty of space, so that you can check when you reach these goals and think about setting yourself some new ones!

This is your book, so fill it in however you like, as long as you do it in a way that means something to you...

Index

"Stand with your fears,
don't hide behind them"

Something beginning with me...

Chapter 1:
'Who I am...'

About me...

Name:

Todays date:

Where I got this book:

My family call me:

My friends call me:

Date of birth:

Star sign*:

Which means...

Born in the Chinese year* of:

Which means...

*see useful stuff on page 152-153

Nationality:

Religion:

Political beliefs:

Who I love:

My best friend:

My girlfriend/boyfriend:

My other friends:

Who inspires me:

My heroes/heroines:

If I wasn't me I'd like to be:

Height:

Weight:

Hair colour:

Eye colour:

Tattoos/piercings:

Distinguishing marks/features:

My other measurements/clothes sizes:

I am: heterosexual/bi-sexual/gay

A virgin - yes / no (where & when...)

Sexually monogamous/sexually adventurous

The thing I like most about myself is:

If there was one thing I could change about myself it
would be:

What I look like:

My hair colour, length and style, eye colour, clothes I wear everyday, clothes I choose to wear for special occasions, or when I'm relaxing. My favourite clothes, shoes, jeans, jewellery, bags, trainers etc...

I would describe myself as...

My family:

My mother, father, step-mother, step-father, carer, foster-parents, brothers and sisters, half-brothers and sisters, grandparents, great-grand parents, aunties, uncles, cousins, nephews & neices, sons & daughters who are important to me...

My family:

Who I am like from the people I have listed and who I am not like and why...

I am like:

Because:

I am not like:

Because:

Recent photographs of me, my family and my friends:

Recent photographs of me, my family and my friends:

Recent photographs of me, my family and my friends:

My 21st birthday celebration...

How I celebrated my 21st birthday and who I did this with.

Where we went:

Who was there:

What we did:

Who helped me plan:

What I was drinking / smoking / taking:

What went better than planned:

What didn't go exactly to plan:

What time I got to bed:

My 21st birthday mood board:

Use the next few pages to create a mood board for your 21st birthday - this might include pictures, tickets, passes, photographs, cards, tags, cut-outs, adverts and other reminders of your celebrations...

My 21st birthday mood board:

My 21st birthday mood board:

My 21st birthday mood board:

"A journey of a thousand miles, starts with a single step"

Something beginning with me...

Chapter 2:
'Where you'll find me...'

Where you'll find me:...

Where I spend my time, places I visit, places I stay and places I travel to on a regular basis...

Where I live:

I have lived here since:

Where else I live from time to time:

A bit about my home:

The kind of place I live in, the size, the number of rooms, bedrooms, bathrooms, garden etc.

Who lives here with me - family, friends and pets:

Other close family who don't live here with me are:

Where they live and how far away this is:

How often I see them and how I get there:

The area we live in:

My local area, its size and surrounding area, the kind of people who live here, and how I get on with them.

Where I lived before:

What it was like, how long I lived there, how it was like / not like where I live now and why:

Where I work:

Name of my employer:

Address:

I've been working here since:

Kind of business:

Number of offices/sites/shops:

My job title:

What I do:

Who I get on with at work:

How I get to and from work:

How long this takes:

How much I earn per week/month:

What I spend my money on:

Where I go to University:

I have been studying here since:

I am studying:

Who I live/hang out with:

Where we hang out most of the time:

What I like about University:

What I don't like about University

How often I go home and how I get there:

Virtual places you'll find me:

My favourite on-line networks, sites and games, how much time I spend on these and who I meet or talk to there...

	use this (yes/no)	who I talk to this way:
e-mail		
mobile phone		
text (phone)		
skype		
facebook		
msn/ windows live		
twitter		
myspace		
bbm		
nintendo		
google +		
playstation		
steam		
other...		

Where else you'll find me:

Family and friends' homes, outdoor places, gym, parks, clubs, classes, cinemas, church, shops, restaurants, fast-food joints, museums, galleries, sports grounds etc.

How I get around between these places...

How long I have been driving/riding:

Where I learned:

How many lessons & how long I took:

How much this cost:

I passed my test on ____ attempt

Reasons for test failure (if appropriate:

What I drive/ride..

Make:

Model:

Registration:

Colour:

Value:

Annual insurance:

Modifications/improvements I have made:

My dream* vehicle:

Realistic goal* for my next vehicle:

*set yourself a goal to achieve this on chapter 6

Where I spend my time:

This is a pie chart* of how much time I spend at each of these places per week.

Each slice is about 10.5 hours of time...

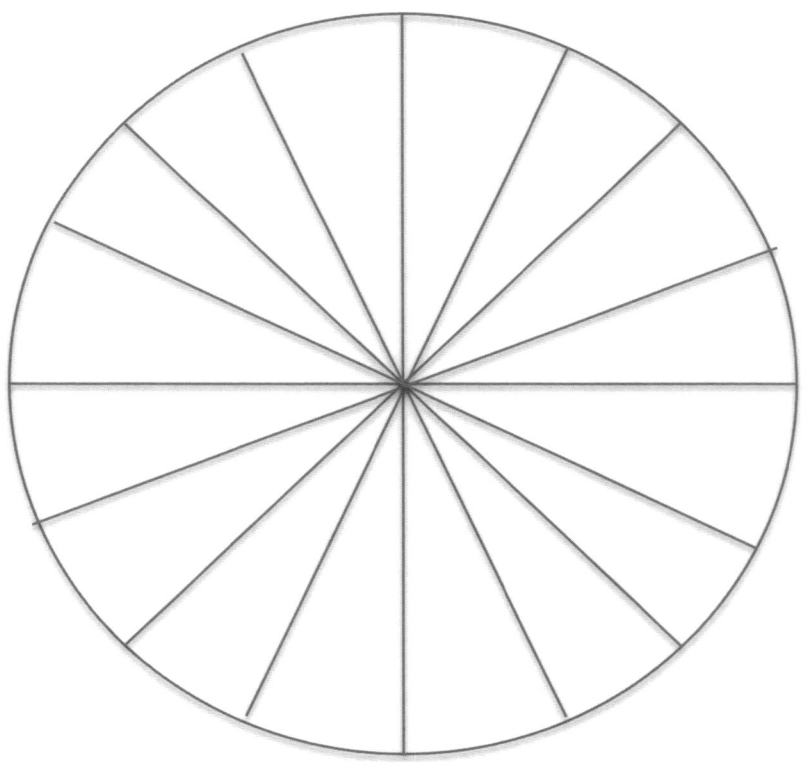

*see pages 148-149

This is how much time I would **like** to spend at each of these places per week...

Each slice is about 10.5 hours of time...

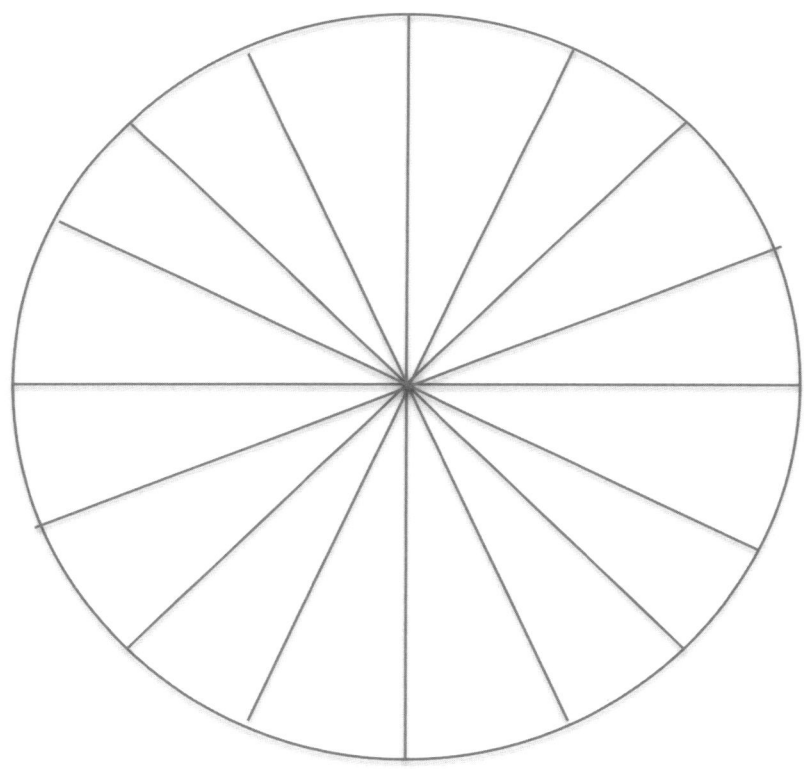

Go to chapter 6 to set yourself some goals to achieve this

Holidays:

What I did during my holidays this year and who I did this with:

Where we went and how we got there:

Where we stayed:

How long we stayed for

Things I did and if I'd like to do these again sometime:

Best thing/s about this holiday:

What didn't go to plan:

or... I didn't go on holiday this year because...

Photographs and other reminders of my most recent holiday:

Photographs and other reminders of my most recent holiday:

Places* I have been...

Places* I have been, but would not choose to go back to...

*See pages 138-141 for a list of countries of the world in aphabetical order

46

Places* I would like to go one day...

"always do your best -
what you plant now, you
will harvest later"

Og Mandino

Something beginning with me...

Chapter 3:
'Things I do...'

The things you'll see me doing...

Things I like to do and those I don't, on my own and with other people:

If I have time to myself, I like to...

I'm very good at...

I'm not so good at...

Relaxing:

Things I like to do when I am not studying, working or looking after others; my favourite sports, games, hobbies, interests, web sites, supporting sports teams, etc:

Things I do to relax, chillout and wind down:

Things that I don't like having to do and what I do to avoid these if possible:

things I do to prepare myself to do these things:

Use chapter 6 to set yourself some goals/targets in this area

Listening to things:

My favourite music, songs, radio shows, bands, groups, musicians etc:

Things I don't like having to listen to and why:

My top 10 songs/tracks right now:

	track or song	artist/band
1		
2		
3		
4		
5		
6		
7		
8		
9		
10		

My top 10 songs / tracks of all time:

	track or song	artist / band
1		
2		
3		
4		
5		
6		
7		
8		
9		
10		

Watching:

Things I like to watch - tv programmes, youtube, films, sports, cartoons, activities, comedy, theatre:

People I like to watch - my favourite people, groups, comedians, celebrities, politicians, tv presenters, athletes, sports teams etc...:

Things I don't like having to watch and why:

Top 10 TV programmes right now:

	title	why I like it...
1		
2		
3		
4		
5		
6		
7		
8		
9		
10		

Top 10 TV programmes of all time:

	title	why I like it...
1		
2		
3		
4		
5		
6		
7		
8		
9		
10		

Top 10 films of all time:

	title	why I like it/ best scenes/lines
1		
2		
3		
4		
5		

	title	why I like it/ best scenes/lines
6		
7		
8		
9		
10		

Reading:

Things that I like to read and why, including my favourite books, comics, magazines, journals, blogs, newspapers, websites, tweets etc:

Things I don't like having to read and why:

Favourite books, authors & characters:

	book/author/ character	why
1		
2		
3		
4		
5		

	book/author/character	why
6		
7		
8		
9		
10		

Eating and drinking:

My favourite foods, snacks, treats, restaurants, take-aways etc:

My favourite diet:

Things I don't like to eat or drink and why:

Foods and drinks I've never tried but would like to try one day:

Things I like to cook, make or prepare and my
favourite recipes/chefs/cooks:

Last meal I cooked for someone else:

Date:

Who:

Why:

What I cooked:

How long this took:

Overall marks for this event   /10

"Don't walk behind me; I may not lead. Don't walk infront of me; I may not follow. Just walk beside me and be my friend. "

Albert Camus

Something beginning with me...

Chapter 4:
'Who I know...'

Who you'll see me with...

These are the people that I see and talk with most often. Some of them I like more than others, some make me laugh and make me happy, others annoy and frustrate me!

Use chapter 6 to set yourself some goals/targets in this area

who/ relationship	what I think about them/how they make me feel...

who/ relationship	what I think about them/how they make me feel...

Who you'll see me with...

This is a mind map* of the people I spend my time with.

* see pages 150-151

Using the map that I've drawn, these are the people that I'd like to spend more time with, to talk with more or to get closer to and some ideas about how I can to do this...

name	what I'm going to do...	when...

name	what I'm going to do...	when...

Relationships...

My ideal type:

Male/female:

Build:

Hair colour:

Eye colour:

Skin colour:

Nationality:

Political views:

Personality type:

Piercings/tatoos etc.:

Other characteristics/attributes:

My current/last boyfriend/girlfriend:

Name:

Age:

Height:

Weight:

Hair colour:

Eye colour:

Skin colour:

Nationality:

Tattoos/piercings:

Other distinguishing marks/features:

I'd describe them as:

What I love/loved about them:

What frustrated/s me about them:

Who I miss:

As we get older there are people who move away and we lose contact with, or people and pets who die.

These are some of the people/pets who I no longer see and why I miss them...

These are some of the things I can do to remember them when I need to:

This is how I can contact them if I need to:

Who I go to for help:

Certain people help us maybe with advice, ideas, comfort or cheering-up. They make us laugh, listen to our problems, share our concerns or help us to celebrate our successes.

When I need something these are the people I go to and what I go to them for:

If I want to find out something I will ask/go to:

Where I go to make new friends/contacts:

There are lots of places we can go to find new friends and people who share our interests and hobbies, or to meet with our existing friends.

These are the ways and places I go to do this:

Where I go to make new friends/contacts:

Use chapter 6 to set yourself some goals/targets in this area

"Health is the greatest posession, contentment is the greatest treasure, confidence is the greatest friend, non-being is the greatest joy"

Lau Tzu

Something beginning with
me...

Chapter 5:
'More about me...'

Things I'm good at:

These are some of the things I am good at or that I know about. There are lots of things that I do well and there are also things that I have to work at, but really enjoy doing anyway:

These are some of the things that I am learning to do and how I'm getting on with them, including goals that I've set myself in improving these new skills, talents or abilities:

Things I'm not good at:

These are the things that I don't like doing, or will avoid having to do if possible:

Use chapter 6 to set yourself some goals/targets in this area

My 'best day ever':

If I could plan my best day ever, this is who would be there, what I'd be doing, what the other people would be doing, and why:

My 'worst day ever':

If I had to think of my worst day ever, this is who would be there, what we'd be doing, what I'd find boring, annoying, frustrating etc. and why:

Things that are important to me:

These are some of my favourite posessions; pc, bike, car, games consoles, tv, phone, jewellery, clothes etc and why they are important to me:

thing...	why...

thing...	why...

Things that I believe:

I should...

I ought to...

I must remember to...

It would be good if other people...

It's really important that we...

It's not good to...

The world would be a better place if...

If only I could...

Then...

When I get older it will be important for me to...

When I am older it will mean that I am able to...

Having my own place means I will be able to:

My friends are important to me because...

My family is important to me because...

My health/fitness is importnant to me because...

My finances are important to me because...

It's important for me to be able to...

It's important for me to have...

If only others would...

then...

Things that are important to me:

We all value different things in life, when we value something and it is important to us, we will try to do things that make sure that we get more of these. There are also things which are not important to us and we don't care if we have them or not. These are the 5 things that are most important for me.

values:

acceptance · activity · admiration · appearances · approval · attention · authority · beauty · caring · challenge · cleanliness · collaboration · communication · competition · co-operation · courage · creativity · dignity · difference · education · efficiency · entertainment · equality · excellence · excitement · expression · fairness · faith · fame · family · freedom · friends · fitness · fun · grace · happiness · harmony · health · helping · honesty · image · independence · integrity · insight · innovation · joy · justice · knowledge · learning · logic · looks · love · manners · obedience · order · others · pain avoidance · partnership · peace · perseverance · popularity · power · quiet · reality · reason · recognition · revolution · rewards · respect · relationships · responsibility · religion · safety · security · self-reliance · self-sacrifice · serenity · sharing ·

silence · simplicity · space · style · spirited ·
status · success · time · tolerance · truth ·
trust · uniqueness · variety · vitality ·
wealth · winning · wisdom · zest ·

top 5 things that are most important to me:
1
2
3
4
5

Because these are important to me, I will...

Things I've done that I'm proud of:

recently:

this year:

as far back as I can remember:

Things that I'm not proud of:

recently:

this year:

as far back as I can remember:

I feel most confident when...

The people who help me feel most confident are:

I lack confidence when...

The people who make me feel less confident are:

Use chapter 6 to set yourself some goals/targets in this area

"The biggest adventure
you can take is to live the
life of your dreams"

Oprah Winfrey

Something beginning with me...

Chapter 6:
'My goals, dreams
and targets...'

The questions on the following pages will help you think more about your goals, dreams and targets as you come of age.

As you look back at how you have completed the book, you may decide to set yourself some goals in some or all of the following areas:

- Work goals
- Personal health
- Relationships
- Money
- Learning/self development
- Spiritual life
- Hobbies/interests
- Fun/recreation

Alternatively you might find the list on page 158 a useful checklist of problems that you'd like to tackle.

Take your time to think about how you answer these questions...

What I want to be/what I want to do when I am 30:

	My dreams/goals/targets	How and where I want to do this
1		
2		
3		

Goal/dream/target number: 1 - when I am 30

My goal/dream/target written in **positive** words
(what I want to have, not what I don't want to have!!)

Why this is important to me...

I want to achieve this by...

I want to be able to do this when I am...

When I have achieved this other people will see me...

They will hear me...

I will feel...

To achieve this I will have to...

When I achieve this, I may have to stop...

Because...

To achieve this I will need to learn how to...

I will need help from...

I will need them to help me to...

When I achieve this, my next goal will be to...

Today I will make a start on this goal, bytaking this one small step - I will...

Goal/dream/target number: 2 - when I am 30

My goal/dream/target written in **positive** words
(what I want to have, not what I don't want to have!!)

Why this is important to me...

I want to achieve this by...

I want to be able to do this when I am...

When I have achieved this other people will see me...

They will hear me...

I will feel...

To achieve this I will have to...

When I achieve this, I may have to stop...

Because...

To achieve this I will need to learn how to...

I will need help from...

I will need them to help me to...

When I achieve this, my next goal will be to...

Today I will make a start on this goal, bytaking this one small step - I will...

Goal/dream/target number: 3 - when I am 30

My goal/dream/target written in **positive** words
(what I want to have, not what I don't want to have!!)

Why this is important to me...

I want to achieve this by...

I want to be able to do this when I am...

When I have achieved this other people will see me...

They will hear me...

I will feel...

To achieve this I will have to...

When I achieve this, I may have to stop...

Because...

To achieve this I will need to learn how to...

I will need help from...

I will need them to help me to...

When I achieve this, my next goal will be to...

Today I will make a start on this goal, bytaking this
one small step - I will...

What I want to be/do when I am 25:

	my dreams/goals/targets	how and where I want to do this
1		
2		
3		

Goal/dream/target number: 1 - when I am 25

My goal/dream/target written in **positive** words
(what I want to have, not what I don't want to have!!)

Why this is important to me...

I want to achieve this by...

I want to be able to do this when I am...

When I have achieved this other people will see me...

They will hear me...

I will feel...

To achieve this I will have to...

When I achieve this, I may have to stop...

Because...

To achieve this I will need to learn how to...

I will need help from...

I will need them to help me to...

When I achieve this, my next goal will be to...

Today I will make a start on this goal, bytaking this one small step - I will...

Goal/dream/target number: 2 - when I am 25

My goal/dream/target written in **positive** words
(what I want to have, not what I don't want to have!!)

Why this is important to me...

I want to achieve this by...

I want to be able to do this when I am...

When I have achieved this other people will see me...

They will hear me...

I will feel...

To achieve this I will have to...

When I achieve this, I may have to stop...

Because...

To achieve this I will need to learn how to...

I will need help from...

I will need them to help me to...

When I achieve this, my next goal will be to...

Today I will make a start on this goal, bytaking this one small step - I will...

Goal/dream/target number: 3 - when I am 25

My goal/dream/target written in **positive** words
(what I want to have, not what I don't want to have!!)

Why this is important to me...

I want to achieve this by...

I want to be able to do this when I am...

When I have achieved this other people will see me...

They will hear me...

I will feel...

To achieve this I will have to...

When I achieve this, I may have to stop...

Because...

To achieve this I will need to learn how to...

I will need help from...

I will need them to help me to...

When I achieve this, my next goal will be to...

Today I will make a start on this goal, bytaking this one small step - I will...

What I want to be/what I want to do for me now:

	my dreams/goals/targets	how and where I want to do this
1		
2		
3		

	my dreams/goals/targets	how and where I want to do this
4		
5		
6		

Goal/dream/target number: 1 - for me now:

My goal/dream/target written in **positive** words
(what I want to have, not what I don't want to have!!)

Why this is important to me...

I want to achieve this by...

I want to be able to do this when I am...

When I have achieved this other people will see me...

They will hear me...

I will feel...

To achieve this I will have to...

When I achieve this, I may have to stop...

Because...

To achieve this I will need to learn how to...

I will need help from...

I will need them to help me to...

When I achieve this, my next goal will be to...

Today I will make a start on this goal, bytaking this one small step - I will...

Goal/dream/target number: 2 - for me now

My goal/dream/target written in positive words
(what I want to have, not what I don't want to have!!)

Why this is important to me...

I want to achieve this by...

I want to be able to do this when I am...

When I have achieved this other people will see me...

They will hear me...

I will feel...

To achieve this I will have to...

When I achieve this, I may have to stop...

Because...

To achieve this I will need to learn how to...

I will need help from...

I will need them to help me to...

When I achieve this, my next goal will be to...

Today I will make a start on this goal, bytaking this
one small step - I will...

Goal/dream/target number: 3 - for me now

My goal/dream/target written in **positive** words
(what I want to have, not what I don't want to have!!)

Why this is important to me...

I want to achieve this by...

I want to be able to do this when I am...

When I have achieved this other people will see me...

They will hear me...

I will feel...

To achieve this I will have to...

When I achieve this, I may have to stop...

Because...

To achieve this I will need to learn how to...

I will need help from...

I will need them to help me to...

When I achieve this, my next goal will be to...

Today I will make a start on this goal, bytaking this
one small step - I will...

Goal/dream/target number: 4 - for me now

My goal/dream/target written in **positive** words
(what I want to have, not what I don't want to have!!)

Why this is important to me...

I want to achieve this by...

I want to be able to do this when I am...

When I have achieved this other people will see me...

They will hear me...

I will feel...

To achieve this I will have to...

When I achieve this, I may have to stop...

Because...

To achieve this I will need to learn how to...

I will need help from...

I will need them to help me to...

When I achieve this, my next goal will be to...

Today I will make a start on this goal, bytaking this one small step - I will...

Goal/dream/target number: 5 - for me now

My goal/dream/target written in **positive** words
(what I want to have, not what I don't want to have!!)

Why this is important to me...

I want to achieve this by...

I want to be able to do this when I am...

When I have achieved this other people will see me...

They will hear me...

I will feel...

To achieve this I will have to...

When I achieve this, I may have to stop...

Because...

To achieve this I will need to learn how to...

I will need help from...

I will need them to help me to...

When I achieve this, my next goal will be to...

Today I will make a start on this goal, bytaking this one small step - I will...

Goal/dream/target number: 6 - for me now

My goal/dream/target written in **positive** words
(what I want to have, not what I don't want to have!!)

Why this is important to me...

I want to achieve this by...

I want to be able to do this when I am...

When I have achieved this other people will see me...

They will hear me...

I will feel...

To achieve this I will have to...

When I achieve this, I may have to stop...

Because...

To achieve this I will need to learn how to...

I will need help from...

I will need them to help me to...

When I achieve this, my next goal will be to...

Today I will make a start on this goal, bytaking this one small step - I will...

When I have achieved all of my dreams, goals and targets...

it will be...

I will feel...

you will see me...

144

It will show...

Others will say...

My next steps will be to...

"Do what you love and the necessary resources will follow"

Peter McWilliams

Something beginning with me...

'Useful stuff...'

How to do a pie chart

On pages 40-41 you can do pie charts of where you spend your time. This is a simple way of showing how much of your time you spend on differnt things.

If you imagine the whole pie is 100% of your time and there are 168 hours in a week. If you spend half of your time on one activity and the other half on another, then you would draw a line down the middle of the pie to show 50% on each side (84 hours).

It's more likely that you spend your time on lots of different things and you can estimate how big a slice to allow using these guidelines.

hours	segments of pie
63 hours	6
52.5 hours	5
42 hours	4
31.5 hours	3
21 hours	2
10.5 hours	1
5 hours	0.5

Example pie chart

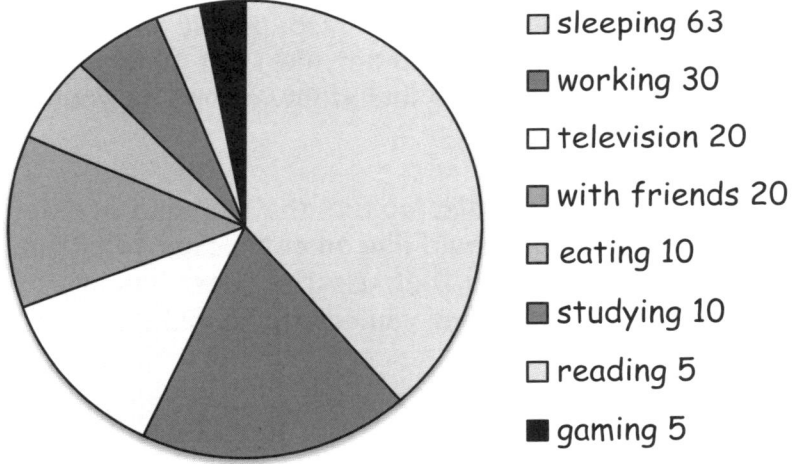

☐ sleeping 63
■ working 30
☐ television 20
■ with friends 20
☐ eating 10
■ studying 10
☐ reading 5
■ gaming 5

How to draw a mind map

On pages 82-83 you will draw a mind map of people you have listed on pages 80-81.

Put your own name in a bubble at the centre of the map and then add in the people in the list by adding each of their names in a bubble.

The closer they are to you, the closer you put their bubble to your bubble on your map, people who are not close to you (or who you do not like) put further away from your bubble. Try to include everyone on your list of contacts.

Once you have done this, look at the map and decide if there is anyone you would like to get closer to or move further away from and then use the questions in chapter 6 to decide what you can do to make this happen.

Your completed map might look something like this...

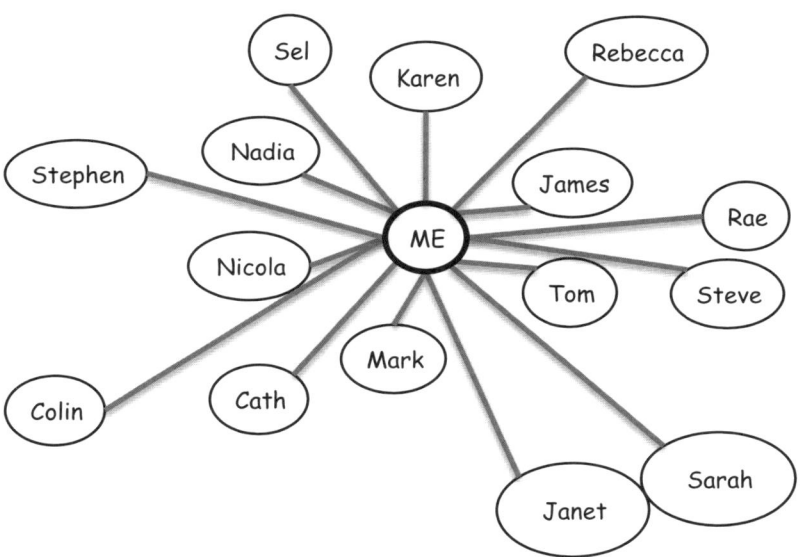

Star signs

Birthday	Your star sign
March 21st - April 19th	Aries
April 20th - May 20th	Taurus
May 21st - June 20th	Gemini
June 21st - July 22nd	Cancer
July 23rd - August 22nd	Leo
August 23rd - September 22nd	Virgo
September 23rd - October 22nd	Llibra
October 23rd - November 21st	Scorpio
November 22nd - December 21st	Sagittarius
December 22nd - January 19th	Capricorn
January 20th - February 18th	Aquarius
February 19th - March 20th	Pisces

Chinese years

The Chinese Lunar calendar names each of the twelve years after an animal.
Legend has it that the Lord Buddha summoned all the animals to come to him before he departed from earth. Only twelve came to bid him farewell and as a reward he named a year after each one in the order they arrived.
The Chinese believe the animal ruling the year in which a person is born is the animal that hides in your heart.

Rat	1948	1960	1972	1984	1996	2008
Ox	1949	1961	1973	1985	1997	2009
Tiger	1950	1962	1974	1986	1998	2010
Rabbit	1951	1963	1975	1987	1999	2011
Dragon	1952	1964	1976	1988	2000	2012
Snake	1953	1965	1977	1989	2001	2013
Horse	1954	1966	1978	1990	2002	2014
Sheep	1955	1967	1979	1991	2003	2015
Monkey	1956	1968	1980	1992	2004	2016
Rooster	1957	1969	1981	1993	2005	2017
Dog	1958	1970	1982	1994	2006	2018
Boar	1959	1971	1983	1995	2007	2019

Countries of the world...

Afghanistan	Bhutan	Cook Islands
Akrotiri	Bolivia	Coral Sea Isles
Albania	Bosnia	Costa Rica
Algeria	Botswana	Cote d'Ivoire
Andorra	Brazil	Croatia
Angola	Brunei	Cuba
Anguilla	Bulgaria	Cyprus
Antartica	Burkina Faso	Czech Republic
Antigua	Burma	Denmark
Argentina	Burundi	Dhekelia
Armenia	Cambodia	Djibouti
Aruba	Cameroon	Dominica
Australia	Canada	Dom Replublic
Austria	Cape Verde	Ecaudor
Azerbaijan	Cayman Islands	Egypt
Bahamas	Central Africa	El Salvador
Bahrain	Chad	Equatorial G'nea
Bangladesh	Chile	Eritrea
Barbados	China	Estonia
Belarus	Christmas Isle	Ethiopia
Belgium	Cocos Islands	Eurpoa Island
Belize	Columbia	Falklands
Benin	Comoros Congo	Faroe Islands
Bermuda	Congo Republic	Fiji

Countries of the world		
Finland	Hong Kong	Laos
France	Hungary	Latvia
French Guiana	Iceland	Lebanon
Fr'ch Polynesia	India	Lesotho
Gabon	Indonesia	Liberia
Gambia	Iran	Libya
Gaza Strip	Iraq	Liechtenstein
Georgia	Ireland	Lithuania
Germany	Isle of Man	Luxembourg
Ghana	Israel	Macau
Gibraltar	Italy	Macedonia
Glorioso Isles	Jamaica	Madagascar
Greece	Jan Mayen	Malawi
Greenland	Japan	Malaysia
Grenada	Jersey	Maldives
Guadeluope	Jordan	Mali
Guam	Juan de Nova	Malta
Guatemala	Kazakhstan	Marshall Isles
Guernsey	Kenya	Martinique
Guinea	Kiribati	Mauritania
Guinea-Bissau	Korea North	Mauritius
Guyana	Korea South	Mayotte
Haiti	Kuwait	Mexico
Honduras	Kyrgyzstan	Micronesia

Countries of the world

Moldova	Pananma	Saudi Arabia
Monaco	Papua N'Guinea	Senegal
Mongolia	Paracel Islands	Serbia
Monserrat	Paraguay	Seychelles
Morocco	Peru	Sierra Leone
Mozambique	Philippines	Singapore
Namibia	Pitcairn Islands	Slovakia
Nauru	Poland	Slovenia
Navassa Island	Portugal	Solomon Islands
Nepal	Puerto Rico	Somalia
Netherlands	Qatar	South Africa
New Caledonia	Reunion	South Georgia
New Zealand	Romania	S Sandwich Isle
Nicaragua	Russia	Spain
Niger	Rwanda	Spratly Islands
Nigeria	Saint Helena	Sri Lanka
Niue	StKitts & Nevis	Sudan
Norfolk Island	Saint Lucia	Suriname
N Mariana Isles	Saint Pierre	Svalbard
Norway	Saint Vincent	Swaziland
Oman	Samoa	Sweden
Pakistan	San Marino	Switzerland
Palau	Sao Tome	Syria

Countries of the world		
Taiwan	Turkey	Vatican City
Tajikistan	Turkmenistan	Venezuela
Tanzania	Turks & Caicos	Vietnam
Thailand	Tuvalu	Virgin Islands
Timor-Leste	Uganda	Wake island
Togo	Ukraine	Wales
Tokelau	United Arab Em	Wallis & Futuna
Tonga	United Kingdom	West Bank
Trinidad &	United States	Westn Sahara
Tobago	Uruguay	Yemen
Tromelin Island	Uzbekistan	Zambia
Tunisia	Vanatu	Zimbabwe

Use this list to see where in the world you have already been and to decide where you might like to go at some point in the future...

You may want to set yourself some goals in chapter 6 in order to make sure you get there!

Problem Areas

Sometimes identifying a problem area is a useful first step in setting yourself some realistic goals that will move your thinking from the problem to the solution. This list is a useful prompt before you set yourself some goals in Chapter 6.

Clarity about values	Lack of assertiveness
Difficult relationships	Poor time management
Lack of direction	Negative emotions
Lack of motivation	Depression
Lack of social skills	Failure to achieve
Health problems	Not able to realx/unwind
Fears/phobias	Chronic pains/injury
Lack of money	Too many demands
Trauma	Lack of results
Decision making	Addiction
Creativity	Lack of confidence
Problem solving	Overworking
Bad habits	Body image/issues
Reoccuring problems from your past	Over-commitment to others

Everything you have written in this book is a way of recording where you are in your life, and where you would like to be. You will have had the opportunity to write down your goals, thoughts, ideas and dreams and this will help you begin to understand more about what's important to you, as you become 21.

Recording the things that you enjoy and the things that annoy you will help you identify the things that you'd like to carry on doing and the things you'd like to change as you grow.

Now that you have filled it in, the book will become a keepsake for you to look back at in the future to help you to remember just how you felt and what you were hoping for at this time. It'll help you to keep track of and remember the story of your amazing life in words, pictures, places, music and songs...

To find out more about 'something beginning with me' and other books in the series, visit our web-site:

www.sbwm.co

Other books in the series:
'something beginning with me...

as I start secondary school

as I become a teenager

at 18

as I start my first job

as I move into my first home

as I get married